Transform Your Family Dynamic: Mastering Parental Anger for a Loving Home!

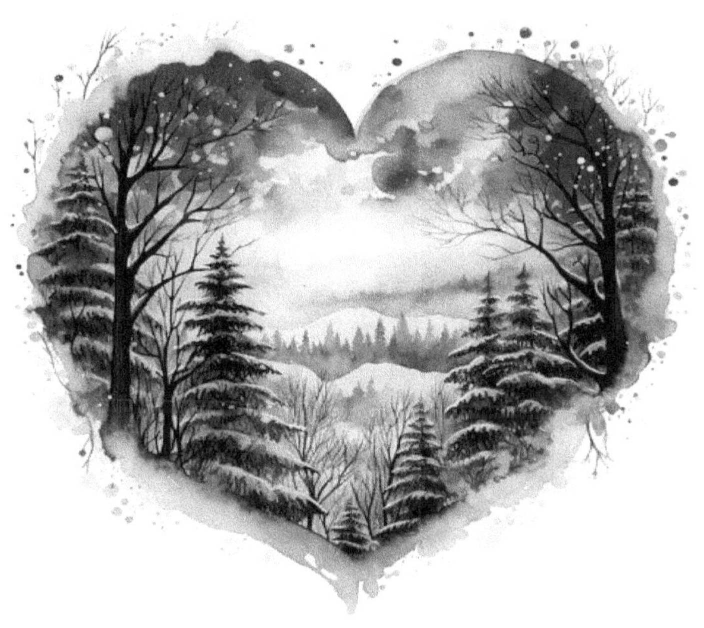

Charles N. Patton

TABLE OF CONTENT

PREFACE

Welcome to "Parenting with Heart"! This book is a heartfelt companion for parents embarking on the rewarding journey of raising children. Filled with practical insights, empathy, and encouragement, it's designed to support you through the ups and downs of parenthood.

As a parent myself, I understand the joys, challenges, and uncertainties that come with the territory. Through personal experiences, research, and the wisdom of experts, this book offers guidance on navigating the complexities of parenting with love, intention, and grace.

Whether you're seeking advice on communication, discipline, self-care, or fostering resilience in your children, "Parenting with Heart" is here to help. May it serve as a beacon of light on your parenting journey, reminding you that you're not alone and that every moment is an opportunity for growth and connection.

Thank you for joining me on this adventure. Together, let's parent with heart and create a nurturing environment where our children can thrive.

Warm regards,

[Charles N. Patton]

Introduction

Establishing a peaceful home environment requires an understanding of the mechanics of rage in parenting. It entails realizing how quickly feelings of tension or annoyance can intensify. Anger can stem from some things, including fatigue, feeling overburdened, or having expectations not realized.

Parents who are aware of these triggers are better able to control their emotions and react composedly in difficult circumstances. With this knowledge, individuals can discern when they must step back and engage in self-care. It also aids in parents' ability to interact with their kids healthily and educate them on how to handle disagreements and emotions.

Families may foster empathy, tolerance, and respect by learning about the dynamics of anger in parenting, which will help them create a caring and loving environment where everyone feels appreciated and understood.

It entails exploring the different causes of parental rage and how it impacts family relationships. Some of these include the following:

Anger triggers can come from a range of causes for parents, such as unresolved personal concerns, stress from job or finances, sleep deprivation, or a sense of being overburdened with duties.

Identifying these stressors is the first step toward controlling your anger.

- Emotional Control: When confronted with difficult circumstances, parents must learn how to control their emotions. This entails being conscious of their emotions, comprehending the reasons behind them, and deciding how to react positively in place of acting rashly and angrily.
- Communication: Handling conflicts and disagreements within the family requires effective communication. In addition to actively listening to their children's

viewpoints, parents should make an effort
to communicate their wants and feelings
aggressively. Transparent and truthful
communication promotes comprehension
and lessens the possibility of
misinterpretations that may result in fury.

- Role Modeling: When it comes to how
  they handle emotions, especially anger,
  parents are extremely influential role
  models for their kids. Since kids pick up
  on their parent's habits, setting a good
  example for them to follow by modeling
  appropriate anger management techniques
  is important. This entails owning up to
  errors, offering regrets when called for,
  and exhibiting compassion and mercy.
- Self-Care: Keeping one's emotional health
  intact requires taking care of oneself, as
  parenting can be taxing at times. Exercise,
  hobbies, and socializing with encouraging
  friends and family are all excellent ways
  for parents to decompress and reenergize
  so they can parent with more resilience
  and patience.

- Seeking Support: When parents are having trouble controlling their anger, it's acceptable for them to do so. This could entail reaching out to a dependable friend or relative, enrolling in a parenting support group, or getting expert assistance from a therapist or counselor with expertise in family dynamics and anger control.

All things considered, recognizing the mechanics of rage in parenting calls for self-awareness, skillful communication, and a dedication to setting an example of appropriate emotional expression for kids. Families may create a loving and supportive atmosphere where everyone feels heard, respected, and loved by managing anger healthily.

Part I: Recognizing Anger Triggers

The Parenting Pressure Cooker: Identifying Stressors

There are moments when being a parent feels like being in a pressure cooker, with stress building up rapidly. Determining what aspects of parenting feel difficult or overwhelming is the first step toward identifying stressors. These pressures might originate from a variety of sources, such as employment, financial concerns, or simply exhaustion from looking after kids all day.

Parents who are aware of these stressors can begin to develop more effective coping mechanisms. This could entail finding ways to unwind and recharge, asking friends or family for assistance, or taking breaks when necessary. Knowing what's stressing them out might help parents learn better-coping mechanisms, which can calm and improve the overall quality of family life.

Let's examine the idea of the "Parenting Pressure Cooker" in more detail and look at stressor identification in a more straightforward way:

Envision a kitchen equipped with a pressure cooker. It builds up pressure till it feels like it might burst when you turn up the heat. In a similar vein, parenting can occasionally feel extremely stressful. Being a parent can involve a lot of strain and stress.

Recognizing stressors entails knowing what they are. For certain parents, it could be the responsibilities of their jobs or financial concerns. Others may experience burnout from tending to kids all day or from handling domestic disputes.

Parents can take action to address these stressors once they are recognized. It's similar to lowering the pressure cooker's heat. This could be learning more effective time management techniques, seeking assistance when required, or figuring out how to unwind and take breaks.

Parents can handle their child's stress by learning what's causing it. This not only makes people feel better, but it also makes the atmosphere at home more peaceful and joyful for both parents and kids.

Unpacking Your Anger: Exploring Root Causes

Finding the source of your anger requires you to delve deep to unpack it, much like when unpacking a suitcase. Investigating the underlying causes of your anger entails going beyond the obvious and figuring out why you're upset in the first place.

Anger can occasionally be likened to an iceberg, with the visible portion representing only a small portion of the deeper issues. Anger in parents is frequently the result of a confluence of elements, such as stress, frustration, unfulfilled demands, and traumatic experiences.

It's crucial to ask yourself the following questions to process your anger:

What had happened just before my outburst? Knowing the instant trigger can help you identify the source of your discomfort.

What's going on below the rage? Anger frequently serves as a cover for more profound emotions like hurt, fear, or grief.

Does my rage follow any pattern? Finding reoccurring events or triggers might assist you in identifying underlying problems that require attention.

What role does my past have in my current anger? Unresolved problems from early life or failed relationships might occasionally be a factor in current rage.

Sincerity and introspection are necessary to investigate the underlying reasons for rage.

Although it's not always simple, this is a crucial first step in improving anger management. Knowing the causes of your anger will help you deal with it head-on and discover healthy outlets for your feelings.

Let's take a closer look at the process of deconstructing your rage and determining its underlying causes:

Thinking Back on Triggers: Begin by thinking back to the events that preceded your anger. Did your youngster say or do anything that caused it? Or was it a tense situation at work or a disagreement with your significant other? Knowing what immediately caused your rage can help you understand what exactly triggered it.

Finding the Hidden Emotions: Anger frequently hides deeper feelings behind the surface. Spend some time thinking about your feelings before the outburst of rage. Did you experience any hurt, disappointment, fear, or overwhelmed? You can more successfully address the underlying reason for your anger if you are aware of the main feeling that is causing it.

Identifying Trends: See if there are any scenarios or triggers that tend to make you angry. This could be specific actions from your kids, particular situations at work, or even encounters with particular individuals. Understanding these patterns can assist you in determining what underlying problems might be causing you to become angry.

Analyzing Past Experiences: Our responses to situations in the present might be influenced by our past experiences, particularly those from our childhood or past relationships. Consider whether your current anger may be a result of unsolved issues or traumas from your past. Investigating these links can bring you important new perspectives on your emotional responses.

Seeking Outside Views: Consulting a therapist, family member, or trusted friend might occasionally be beneficial. They might provide unique viewpoints or insights that you wouldn't have thought of on your own. Sharing your experiences with others can also help to validate and support you emotionally.

How to Exercise Self-Compassion: As you investigate the underlying roots of your rage, keep in mind to treat yourself with kindness. Feeling angry or irritated is acceptable and a normal aspect of the process. Along this path of self-awareness and development, treat yourself with kindness and self-compassion.

You can learn more about yourself and your emotional reactions by exploring the underlying causes of your rage. This knowledge gives you the ability to deal with underlying problems, create healthy coping mechanisms, and foster happier bonds with your family and kids.

Triggers from Childhood: How Your Past Affects Your Present

Childhood triggers can have a significant influence on how we perceive and communicate anger in the present. Our early experiences influence how we relate to others, view the world, and control our emotions. This is how the past can influence the present:

- Acquired Conduct: As children, we watch our parents and other adults manage a range of emotions, including rage. If we grow up seeing someone express their anger in negative ways or with frequent outbursts, we could unintentionally take on similar behavioral patterns as adults.
- Unresolved Trauma: Neglect, abuse, or other types of trauma suffered as a child can leave long-lasting emotional scars. As adults, these unhealed wounds may resurface as sources of rage or other strong emotions, particularly when

confronted with circumstances that evoke the initial trauma.

- Types of Attachments: Our early attachment bonds with our caregivers shape our social interactions and emotional regulation throughout our lives. For instance, people with insecure attachment styles could find it challenging to set appropriate boundaries and control their emotions, which can make it harder to control their anger.
- Fundamental Beliefs: Our worldview and self-perception are shaped by the ideas and messages we assimilate as children. Feelings of invalidation or unworthiness throughout childhood can lead to negative basic beliefs about others and ourselves as adults, which can result in feelings of inadequacy, resentment, or rage.
- Events that Trigger Emotions: As adults, some situations or people might cause intense feelings connected to the past. Repetition: In the absence of awareness and intervention, people may

unintentionally repeat unhealthy patterns of behavior from their childhood in their adult relationships and parenting approaches. These triggers may seem insignificant to others, but they can have a profound emotional resonance for those with unresolved childhood issues, resulting in intense feelings of rage or distress. Interpersonal problems and continuous difficulties with anger might be caused by the continuation of these harmful cycles.

Breaking free from negative habits and building healthier relationships requires an understanding of how your past experiences shape your current reactions. Through compassionate and self-aware exploration of your childhood triggers, you can start to mend old wounds, create useful coping mechanisms, and build a more balanced and meaningful life for your family and yourself.

Let's examine in more detail how childhood triggers may impact your current feelings and outward displays of anger:

- Blueprint for Emotions: Our emotional reactions and coping strategies are shaped by our early experiences. You might carry over some tendencies into your adult life, such as the tendency to express anger explosively or the avoidance of disputes entirely, if you were raised in such a setting. By being aware of this emotional blueprint, you may identify patterns that keep coming up and choose consciously how you want to react to rage right now.

- Unconscious Triggers: Events that occur throughout childhood may leave behind unconscious triggers that, as adults, bring on intense emotional emotions. For example, situations that arouse sentiments of rejection in your adult relationships may cause strong anger or anxiety if you were rejected or abandoned as a child. These triggers have the power to significantly affect your emotional reactions, even if they could be subtle and not always obvious at first.

- Effect on Relationships: How you handle relationships as a youngster might influence how you connect with people as an adult. For instance, you could find it difficult to communicate your anger in adult relationships if you grew up witnessing conflict avoidance or passive-aggressive conduct in your family. On the other hand, if you are prone to confrontation or aggression, you can discover that you respond defensively or violently to people who are angry with you.
- Self-Perception and Worthiness: Your sense of worthiness and self-perception are also influenced by the events of your early years. If you experience criticism, belittling, or invalidation as a child, you can internalize these negative signals and come to believe that you are unworthy or have poor self-esteem. Because of this,

you can be more prone to experiencing emotions like rage, annoyance, or resentment when you think you're being treated unfairly or disrespectfully.

- Recuperation and Development: The first step to recovery and development is realizing how your current experiences of rage are influenced by early triggers. You can learn better-coping strategies and communication techniques by exploring and processing these triggers with the use of therapy, introspection, and mindfulness exercises. You can develop better self-awareness, emotional resilience, and empathy by resolving unresolved issues from your past. This can lead to more rewarding relationships and a stronger sense of well-being in the present.

You can start to break free from ingrained habits and develop more positive ways of relating to both yourself and other people by realizing how your prior experiences have shaped your current sensations of rage. You can develop stronger emotional resilience, empathy, and compassion in your relationships with others around you and yourself by embarking on this path of self-discovery and healing.

Part II: Strategies for Managing Anger

Mindfulness Techniques: Cultivating Awareness and Presence

Developing awareness and presence in the present moment via mindfulness practices can be a strong tool for properly regulating anger.

Here are some benefits of mindfulness:

- Awareness of Triggers: Being mindful entails being aware of your feelings, ideas, and physical experiences without passing judgment. You can learn to recognize the early warning signals of anger, such as tenseness in your body, racing thoughts, or a rapid heartbeat, by engaging in mindfulness practices. You can identify rage triggers early on thanks to this increased awareness, which also empowers you to respond more purposefully and clearly.
- Pause and React: Being mindful enables you to give stimuli and reactions some

distance from one another. You can choose to respond to anger consciously by pausing, taking a few deep breaths, and then acting on your impulses. You can use this time to reflect on other viewpoints and connect with your inner wisdom, which will help you respond to difficult circumstances with greater competence and compassion.

- Emotional Control: Mindfulness techniques, like body scan meditation or mindful breathing, can help you control your emotions and soothe your nervous system. You can anchor yourself in the here and now by focusing on the here and now. This can lessen the intensity of your anger and provide room for more composed and helpful reactions.
- Non-reactivity: You can develop a state of non-reactivity to challenging emotions like rage by practicing mindfulness. You may watch anger with compassion and interest instead of letting it carry you away because you know that feelings are

ephemeral and fleeting occurrences. By adopting this non-reactive attitude, you can respond to anger without being swayed by irrational feelings and instead handle it from a point of inner stability and calm.

- Mindfulness promotes self-compassion and introspection, which enables you to investigate the root causes of your anger with kindness and inquiry. This leads to compassionate self-reflection. You can approach your anger with kindness and understanding, realizing that it's a normal human emotion, rather than with severe self-judgment or placing blame. By practicing compassionate self-reflection, you can develop increased emotional intelligence and resilience, which will help you grow and learn from your experiences.

Mindfulness activities facilitate the development of empathy and connection with others by encouraging a more profound comprehension of their experiences and viewpoints. You grow more sympathetic to other people's experiences—including those of your kids—as you become more aware of your feelings and responses. Your family feels more connected to one another and supportive of one another as a result of your improved empathy.

You may develop more awareness, present, and emotional resilience by implementing mindfulness practices into your daily routine. This will help you respond to rage in parenting and other contexts with better competence and compassion.

Communication Skills: Assertive Expression and Active Listening

Parenting successfully requires the ability to communicate. Anger management is no exception. Active listening and assertive communication are essential for promoting understanding, settling disputes, and forging closer bonds with your kids. This is where these abilities come in handy:

- Assertive Expression: Being assertive in communication is voicing your needs, wants, and opinions in an honest, polite manner while also honoring the rights and boundaries of others. When you speak assertively, you avoid using violence or passive-aggressiveness to get your point across in a clear, confident manner.
- Expressing Emotions: You can calmly and in control convey your emotions, even rage, by using assertive expression. "I" statements, like "I feel frustrated when...", can help you express your feelings without acting out or repressing them.
- Establishing Boundaries: Being assertive helps you to firmly but gently establish and enforce boundaries with your kids. You create a structure and mutual respect in the parent-child connection by being upfront about your expectations and boundaries.

- Problem-Solving: Open communication and problem-solving are fostered by assertive communication. Rather than waging a power battle or using harsh punishment, you and your kids can collaborate to find answers and deal with the underlying problems that lead to conflict or rage.
- The skill of completely interacting with and comprehending what people are saying without passing judgment or interjecting is known as "active listening." It entails paying close attention to what they are saying, recognizing their point of view, and confirming their emotions.
- Empathetic Understanding: Even when your children's opinions and feelings diverge from your own, you may still sympathize with them by actively listening to them. You may establish a safe space for your children to express themselves honestly and freely by listening to them intently and without passing judgment.

- Clarifying Understanding: To make sure that both parties understand each other, active listening entails summarizing and paraphrasing what has been stated. You can show that you are genuinely listening to them and confirming their experiences by thinking back on what they said and how they felt.
- Developing Trust: Active listening helps to develop trust between parents and children. Even amid conflict or pain, children are more inclined to communicate honestly and ask for their parents' support when they feel heard and understood.

You may foster a more pleasant and encouraging family atmosphere by improving your communication skills, which include aggressive expression and active listening. These abilities help you resolve disagreements with more understanding and empathy, which improves relationships and helps your kids develop emotionally.

Stress Management: Coping Mechanisms for Parents

For parents to preserve their health and successfully navigate the difficulties of parenthood without giving in to rage or exhaustion, stress management is essential. The following are coping strategies that parents might use to reduce stress:

- Self-Care: Make time for self-care practices that support your mental, emotional, and physical well. This can involve doing things you enjoy, such as hobbies or spending time with loved ones, as well as getting enough sleep, eating healthily, and exercising regularly. Taking care of oneself helps you feel more energized and better able to handle the responsibilities of parenthood.
- Techniques for Relaxation and Mindfulness: To relax your body and mind, try progressive muscle relaxation, deep breathing techniques, or mindfulness

meditation. These methods help you de-stress, lower your stress hormone levels, and become more resilient to stressful situations. A daily mindfulness practice of even a few minutes can have a big impact on your stress levels.

- Time management: Create efficient time management plans to arrange chores in order of importance, establish reasonable objectives, and allot time for important activities like job, child care, and leisure activities. Make use of time-blocking strategies, calendars, and to-do lists as tools to help you manage your schedule and feel less overwhelmed.

- Seeking Support: When you're feeling overwhelmed, don't be afraid to ask your partner, your family, or your friends for help. Talking to other people about your thoughts and feelings can offer a sense of companionship, as well as practical support and emotional affirmation. In addition, if you feel that you need professional help, think about attending a parenting support group or consulting a therapist or counselor.

- Establishing Limits: To avoid burnout and preserve balance in your life, set clear boundaries about your time, energy, and responsibilities. Saying no to extra obligations or activities that put your health or well-being at risk is a valuable skill. Give top priority to pursuits that are consistent with your values and enhance your sense of fulfillment and happiness in general.
- Healthy Communication: Effective stress management depends on having honest and open conversations with your partner, kids, and other family members. As you attentively listen to other people's viewpoints, you should also assertively communicate your wants, worries, and feelings. Family ties are strengthened, tensions are decreased, and understanding is fostered via effective communication.
- Take Part in Calm Activities: To decompress and revitalize yourself,

incorporate relaxation techniques into your daily routine. This can be doing yoga, reading a book, listening to music, having a warm bath, or going outside. Taking part in enjoyable and relaxing activities relieves stress and revitalizes the soul.

Parents may develop better resilience, preserve their well-being, and handle the demands of parenting with more ease and grace by putting these stress management coping methods into practice. Recall that taking care of oneself is not selfish; rather, it is a necessary part of being a good parent and fostering positive family dynamics.

Setting Boundaries: Establishing Healthy Limits

Establishing boundaries is crucial for retaining equilibrium, safeguarding well-being, and cultivating positive relationships—particularly when it comes to parenting. Here's how parents can set appropriate boundaries:

- Determine Your Limitations and Needs: Consider your own needs, values, and priorities for a while. Think about the interactions, behaviors, and circumstances that you find acceptable and those that make you uncomfortable or difficult. Setting boundaries that work requires first understanding your limitations.
- Express Yourself Clearly and Firmly: Be calm and firm while expressing your boundaries to your partner, kids, and other family members. Express your needs and preferences with "I" statements, such as "I need some quiet time to recharge" or "I prefer not to be interrupted when I'm working." Establish and maintain boundaries with consistency and firmness.
- Set Boundaries for Time and Energy: To prevent overcommitting or feeling overburdened, set limits for the amount of time and energy you spend. Set priorities

for tasks and commitments that fit with your beliefs and objectives, and develop the ability to refuse offers or demands that are greater than what you can handle.

- Explain Consequences: Explain to them what will happen if they cross your limits. This could be leaving the situation, taking some time out to collect yourself, or imposing a particular punishment for persistently crossing boundaries. Enforcing penalties consistently serves to underscore how important it is to respect limits.
- Establish Healthy Boundaries: Set a good example for your kids by modeling appropriate boundary-setting techniques. In your dealings with other people, exhibit assertive communication, self-respect, and an understanding of the value of self-care. Since kids pick up on behavior from their parents, setting good examples in the form of healthy boundaries for them to follow in their relationships is important.

- Exercise Self-Compassion: While you work through the process of establishing boundaries, treat yourself with kindness and respect. While it's common to experience guilt or anxiety while voicing your demands, keep in mind that putting your health first is crucial for both good parenting and preserving wholesome relationships. Develop self-love and self-compassion to strengthen your emotional fortitude.

- Seek Assistance: If you find it difficult to set or maintain limits, don't be afraid to ask your friends, partner, or therapist for help. Have an honest conversation about your worries and difficulties, and come up with ideas on how to properly create boundaries in different circumstances. Having a solid support system around you might help you negotiate setting boundaries by offering words of wisdom and validation.

Establishing boundaries is a continuous process that calls for consistency, firmness, and self-awareness. Parents foster a loving and courteous home atmosphere where everyone's needs are recognized and met by setting reasonable boundaries. Setting limits effectively encourages mental health, lessens conflict, and builds closer, more satisfying bonds among family members.

Part III: Healing and Growth

Forgiveness and Compassion: Towards Yourself and Your Children

Compassion and forgiveness are effective means of fostering wholesome bonds and advancing mental health in the family. Here are some tips for parents on how to develop compassion and forgiveness for both themselves and their kids:

- Self-forgiveness: Being a parent is a difficult road with many highs and lows, therefore it's normal to make mistakes along the way. To cultivate self-forgiveness, accept your flaws, and let go of shame and self-criticism. Realize that you're making the best effort you can with the information and tools at your disposal, and give yourself permission to develop and learn from your experiences.

- Exercise self-compassion by treating yourself with the same consideration and compassion that you would show a friend going through a comparable situation. When things are tough, remember to be kind to yourself by supporting, affirming, and encouraging yourself. This is a sign of self-compassion. Develop self-awareness and mindfulness to identify instances of self-criticism and to swap out critical self-talk with supportive and encouraging remarks.

- Embrace Imperfection: Recognize that being a parent is a lifelong learning and growth process and that it's acceptable to have imperfections. Accept the untidy, awkward times that come with being a parent with kindness and humor, since they are an essential part of the journey. Let go of the need to be a flawless parent and concentrate on creating a nurturing atmosphere for both you and your kids.

- In your dealings with your kids, set an example of forgiveness and compassion by owning up to your faults and offering an apology. Show humility and vulnerability by owning up to your mistakes and showing sincere regret if you have offended or disappointed your kids. They learn important lessons from this about empathy, responsibility, and the value of mending relationships.

- Encourage Emotional Expression: Provide a secure and nurturing environment where your kids can freely and honestly express their feelings. Even if you disagree with their viewpoint, acknowledge their emotions and show empathy and compassion. When they encounter difficulties or make mistakes, encourage them to be kind and forgiving of themselves.
- Teach Empathy and Understanding: Help your kids develop empathy and understanding by educating them to take into account the thoughts and feelings of others. Encourage your siblings, friends, and classmates to act with love,

compassion, and forgiveness. Assist them
in seeing that forgiveness is a self-gift that
releases them from the weight of grudges
and rage.

- Honor Development and Progress: Honor
the development and advancement you
and your kids experience as you move
closer to compassion and forgiveness.
Acknowledge and value the efforts you're
making to support your family's emotional
wellness and strong relationships.
Celebrate all of your accomplishments, no
matter how minor, and give thanks for
your shared love and bond.

Fostering forgiveness and compassion for both
yourself and your kids helps to build a loving
and encouraging family atmosphere where
everyone is accepted, understood, and feels
important. These attributes fortify links,
encourage emotional forbearance, and cultivate a
feeling of inclusion and closeness among family
members.

Seeking Support: Building a Support Network

Parents need to seek assistance and establish a solid support system to deal with the difficulties of parenting, stress management, and preserving their well-being. Here's how parents can create a network of support:

- Speak with Your Friends and Family: Rely on your friends and family for practical help, encouragement, and emotional support. Tell trusted family members about your struggles, worries, and victories so they can provide you with support, guidance, and a listening ear. Building relationships with friends and family makes people feel connected and like they belong, which promotes resilience and well-being.
- Join Communities or Parenting Groups: Look for online communities, parenting organizations, or support systems where you can get in touch with other parents going through similar struggles. These

groups give people a forum to discuss parenting advice, exchange experiences, and offer support to one another. Joining a parenting group can help you feel less alone, validate yourself, and get insightful knowledge from other parents going through similar experiences.

- Participate in Parenting Courses or Classes: Sign up for online or locally provided parenting courses or classes. These programs offer helpful information, tools, and doable tactics for handling all facets of parenting, from self-care and stress reduction to communication and discipline. By taking part in parenting education, you can enhance your parenting skills and gain confidence in your role as a parent by gaining information and skills.

- Seek Professional Support: If you're having trouble with parenting, relationships, or mental health difficulties, don't be afraid to get help from therapists, counselors, or parenting coaches. A trained specialist can provide tailored advice, resources, and techniques to address particular issues, strengthen communication, and improve coping mechanisms. A secure and private setting is offered by therapy or counseling to explore feelings, gain understanding, and create useful coping strategies for stress management and improving well-being.

- Attend Support Groups or Therapy: Consider enrolling in groups or therapy sessions that are expressly designed to address parenting-related concerns. Examples of these include family therapy, co-parenting support groups, and postpartum support groups. These groups provide a safe space to talk about parenting difficulties, exchange stories, and get advice from peers and experts. Establishing connections with those undergoing comparable circumstances can offer affirmation, insight, and motivation, cultivating a feeling of unity and adaptability.

- Make Use of Internet Resources: Look through blogs, podcasts, and discussion boards devoted to parenting and family support on the Internet. From baby care and toddler discipline to teen parenting and self-care, these resources provide a plethora of knowledge, pointers, and guidance on a range of parenting subjects. You can interact with parents all around the world, gain access to a variety of viewpoints, and get support and inspiration from the comfort of your own home by participating in online groups.
- Prioritize Self-Care: Always remember to give yourself the attention and time you need to engage in things that feed your body, mind, and spirit. Taking care of yourself improves resilience, restores your energy, and makes it possible for you to be a more present and successful parent. Establish limits on your time and responsibilities, assign work when it can be done, and give pleasure and

relaxation-inducing activities a top priority.

Creating a support system is a continuous process that calls for open communication, vulnerability, and work. You may build a network of care and support that helps you deal with the ups and downs of parenting with resilience and confidence by asking for help and connecting with people who can relate to your experiences.

Modeling Emotional Regulation: Teaching by Example

One of the best things parents can do to help their kids learn how to control their emotions is to model emotional regulation. Here are some ways parents can set a good example:

- Acknowledge Your Feelings: To begin with, become conscious of your feelings and how they affect the way you behave. Recognize when you're stressed, frustrated, or furious, and observe your behavior during such times. You can start modeling good emotional regulation for your kids by acknowledging your feelings.
- Pause and Think: Give yourself a moment to stop and think before responding to intense emotions to avoid acting on an impulse. This enables you to collect your ideas, think through the effects of your choices, and select a more positive outlet for your emotions. Teaching kids to pause and think about their decisions helps them learn the value of self-control and deliberate decision-making.
- Express Emotions Calmly: Be assertive and calm when expressing your feelings. Yelling, placing blame, or using harsh language should be avoided as these actions can intensify arguments and impede clear communication. Instead,

model assertive communication and emotional expression for your children by using "I" statements to explain how and why you feel.

- Employ Coping Strategies: Show how to use constructive coping mechanisms to control your emotions and stress. This could be practicing mindfulness meditation, deep breathing techniques, going for a stroll, or doing something creative. You may teach your kids that it's possible to deal with tough emotions in healthy ways by modeling these coping strategies.
- Admit Errors and Offer Apologies: Children must understand that mistakes are made by adults too, since nobody is flawless. If you do snap or respond in a way you later regret, own up to it and provide a heartfelt apology. Children learn from this how important it is to accept accountability for their acts, mend relationships, and grow from their mistakes.

- Promote the Expression of Emotions:
  Establish a secure and encouraging
  atmosphere that encourages your kids to
  communicate their feelings honestly and
  freely. Pay close attention, acknowledge
  their emotions, and extend understanding
  and unprejudiced support. Children learn
  that it's acceptable to feel and express
  their emotions honestly when adults
  model acceptance of a diverse spectrum of
  emotions.

- Provide Problem-Solving Techniques:
  Teach kids how to solve problems so they
  can deal with the underlying problems that
  are giving them grief, rather than only
  emphasizing emotion management. Assist
  them in pinpointing the cause of their
  feelings, formulating potential fixes, and
  weighing the pros and drawbacks of each
  choice. Giving kids the ability to solve
  problems on their own gives them
  important tools for overcoming obstacles
  in life.

Parents may help their children develop strong interpersonal skills, resilience, and effective emotion management by modeling good coping mechanisms and emotional regulation. Keep in mind that kids pick up the majority of their knowledge from seeing the conduct of the adults in their environment, so make an effort to provide a good example of emotional stability and self-control in your family.

CONCLUSIONS

Embracing Transformation: Moving Forward in Parenting with Awareness and Empathy

Parenting with acceptance of transformation is a path of self-awareness, development, and empathy that encourages constructive change and stronger bonds within the family. Here's how parents can proceed with consciousness and compassion:

1. Develop Self-Awareness: Start by practicing mindfulness, introspection, and reflection to develop self-awareness. Examine your ideas, feelings, and actions, and consider how these affect your interactions with your kids and your parenting style. Understanding your values, triggers, strengths, and limitations will help you make deliberate decisions that support your goals and aspirations as a parent.

2. Parent with awareness: Accept
    mindfulness as the foundation of your
    parenting style. Engage in daily activities,
    talks, and interactions with your children
    by being present and involved.
    Throughout the day, take note of the little
    instances of happiness, connection, and
    education. By promoting acceptance,
    tolerance, and nonjudgmental awareness,
    mindful parenting helps parents and kids
    develop stronger ties and a greater
    capacity for understanding.

3. Embrace Learning and Growth: Develop a
    growth attitude that welcomes obstacles,
    errors, and chances for personal
    development. Consider parenting as a
    lifelong learning process where you
    constantly modify, develop, and hone your
    techniques in light of fresh perceptions
    and encounters. Accept lifelong learning
    and provide an example of
    growth-oriented thinking for your kids.
    This will inspire them to take on

challenges and persevere in the face of failure.

4. Develop Empathy and Compassion: Give these qualities top priority while interacting with your kids and other people. Even in situations where their opinions, feelings, and experiences diverge from your own, try to comprehend and validate them. Acknowledge that being a parent is a difficult and flawed journey and provide empathy to yourself. Emotional intelligence and self-compassion are the cornerstones of fostering kindness and empathy in the family.

5. Encourage Open Communication: Establish an atmosphere that allows people to freely and politely express their ideas, feelings, and concerns. Encourage open communication, attentive listening, and respect for one another among family members. Provide your family with chances for deep dialogue, problem-solving, and conflict resolution

to foster understanding, trust, and a sense of belonging.

6. Accept Adaptability and Flexibility: Accept that being adaptable and flexible is necessary for negotiating the challenges of family life and parenting. Remember that every child is different and might need a different approach or set of concessions. Be prepared to modify your expectations and parenting techniques in response to your child's evolving requirements, developmental stages, and personal preferences.

7. Celebrate Your Progress and Milestones: No matter how tiny, acknowledge and honor the advancements and landmarks you have reached in your parenting career. Celebrate your children's development and achievements while also acknowledging your efforts, maturation, and successes as a parent. Create a joyful, appreciative, and appreciative culture within the family to reinforce good conduct and create a sense of pride and community.

Parents may foster a loving and supportive family environment where everyone feels seen, heard, and valued by accepting change with understanding and sensitivity. The basis for a lifetime of love and understanding is laid by this path of development and connection, which also strengthens the bond between parents and children and promotes resilience and well-being.

"Thank you for embarking on this heartfelt journey with 'Parenting with Heart.' Your dedication to nurturing strong, loving connections within your family is truly inspiring. As you turn the final page, know that your commitment to parenting with intention and compassion is making a profound difference in the lives of those you love most. May the wisdom found within these pages continue to guide you on your path, filling your home with warmth, laughter, and endless love. With heartfelt gratitude, [Charles N. Patton]."

www.ingramcontent.com/pod-product-compliance
Lightning Source LLC
Chambersburg PA
CBHW072340270726
48659CB00022B/2099